Low Fodmap Diet

This Cookbook Will Assist You In Locating The IBS Cure
And Alleviating Digestive Disorder Symptoms

*(How To Begin A Low Fodmap Diet With Simple Gut-
soothing Recipes)*

I0083583

Hans-Günther Liedtke

TABLE OF CONTENT

Introduction

There are numerous diseases with symptoms similar to those of irritable bowel syndrome, so an accurate diagnosis must be made prior to treating this condition and attempting to adhere to a particular diet.

There is currently no universal diet that would be suitable for all patients with irritable bowel syndrome. However, many IBS patients attribute the worsening of their symptoms to certain foods, and excluding these foods from their diet aids in their recovery.

Because there is no universal diet, what works for one individual may not work for another. Your optimal dietary modifications are determined by your specific symptoms and food-related reactions.

A food journal can help you identify foods that alleviate or exacerbate your symptoms. We recommend keeping track of the foods you eat, the symptoms you experience, and the amount of time it takes for the symptoms to manifest after eating.

Chapter 1: The Side Effects Of Eating A Low-Fodmap Diet And The Risks Involved In The Process

Low FODMAP Diet Side Effects & Risks
Following a low-FODMAP diet has been shown to reduce symptoms of irritable bowel syndrome (IBS), but this does not mean the diet is risk-free.

Nutrient Deficiencies
Typically, FODMAP-rich foods are also rich in the vitamins and minerals required by the body. People who do not consume adequate amounts of vitamin D, calcium, iron, zinc, and folate run the risk of developing serious health issues.

This diet phase is the most dangerous because it restricts the consumption of so many different food groups; however, it should only last for a brief period of time to prevent long-term damage. To ensure that nutrient deficiencies do not remain a problem during stages 2 and 6 require consultation with a qualified nutritionist.

Vitality of the Gut Flora

Gut flora must be fed nutrient-rich food to maintain its viability and proliferate. Due to the fact that FODMAPs are the food source for certain beneficial bacteria, such as Bifidobacteria, their populations will decrease when exposed to a low-FODMAP diet.

Butyrate is one of the short-chain fatty acids (SCFAs) produced when beneficial bacteria ferment tiny carbohydrate molecules in the stomach. The cells that line the large intestine are nourished in turn by these cells. Therefore, it is possible that your body requires FODMAPs for optimal function.

If you do not have irritable bowel syndrome (IBS), a low-FODMAP diet may do more harm than good for your gut flora. It is essential to consult a medical professional prior to beginning the diet, which is one reason why.

Difficulties with Maintaining Adherence
Maintaining a diet low in FODMAPs can be difficult, especially in the absence of information or in a social setting. People may not be able to identify the appropriate foods on their own, and restaurants and other social settings are unlikely to label low FODMAP options explicitly.

The most effective strategy for promoting adherence is written and in-person consultation with a qualified professional. People have a much greater chance of successfully adopting a low FODMAP diet if they have reliable access to an expert who can guide them through maintaining diet adherence.

Expenses

Those adhering to a strict FODMAP diet would be required to replace staple foods with pricey alternatives such as exotic fruits and "pseudo-cereals" to prevent nutritional deficiencies (such as amaranth, quinoa, and buckwheat)

Examples of low FODMAP levels in Chapter 2

Daily consumption of FODMAPs from a FODMAP-rich diet or a conventional diet may range from 0.10 to 2 ounce (2 10 to 6 0 grammes) of these carbohydrates.

A low FODMAP diet, on the other hand, aims to limit your consumption to 0.02 ounces (0.10 grammes) per meal, which is an extremely low amount that equates to 0.08–0.2 ounces (2.10 –6 grammes) per day if you adhere to the recommendation of eating several small meals per day.

Fortunately, a wide variety of foods naturally contain low levels of FODMAPs. Following is a list of foods that adherers to a low FODMAP diet are permitted to consume.

High-protein foods consist of beef, chicken, fresh eggs , fish, lamb, pork, prawns, tempeh, and tofu.

Whole grains and starches include white rice, brown rice, lentils, corn, oats, quinoa, cassava, and potatoes.

Fruit examples include blueberries, raspberries, strawberries, pineapple, honeydew melon, cantaloupe, kiwi, limes, guava, starfruit, grapes, and grapefruit.

This dish contains a variety of vegetables, including bean sprouts, bell peppers, radishes, bok choy, carrots, celery, eggplant, kale, tomatoes, spinach, cucumber, pumpkin, and zucchini.

Almonds (no more than ten per session), macadamia nuts, peanuts, pecans, pine nuts, and walnuts are permitted.

Seeds: pumpkin, sesame, and sunflower seeds, as very well as linseeds

Cheeses such as mozzarella, cheddar, Colby, and Parmesan, lactose-free milk, and Greek yoghurt are examples of dairy products.

Various oils, including coconut and olive

We have peppermint tea and water for beverages.

Cumin, saffron, cinnamon, paprika, coriander, cardamom, soy sauce, fish sauce, certain products derived from chilli peppers, ginger, mustard, pepper, salt, white rice vinegar, and wasabi powder are used as seasonings.

On a low FODMAP diet, caffeinated beverages are typically discouraged because caffeine tends to be a trigger for individuals with irritable bowel syndrome (IBS). Even though coffee, black tea, and green tea are considered to be low-FODMAP foods, they should be consumed in moderation.

In addition, it is vital to examine the ingredient lists of prepackaged foods to determine if they contain additional FODMAPs. Manufacturers may add FODMAPs to foods for various purposes, including as prebiotics, low-calorie sugar alternatives, or fat replacements.

Chapter 2: Why Is Digesting Fodmaps So Difficult?

FODMAPs are fermentable short-chain carbohydrate chains. That is equivalent to two things: Because they are chains of sugar molecules, the microorganisms in your stomach are able to ferment them. For chains of molecules to be absorbed by the small intestine, they must be disassembled into individual molecules. FODMAPs cannot be metabolised and therefore cannot be absorbed there. The small intestine absorbs additional water to facilitate the passage of FODMAPs to the large intestine. There, the bacteria in your colon have a field day fermenting them (eating them). This causes your stomach to produce gas and fatty acids as a result.

Are FODMAPs dangerous for everyone?

In no way. In reality, our digestive systems can process foods that we cannot completely digest, such as dietary fibre, which is essential for digestive health. In addition, we feed them as part of our symbiotic relationship with these bacteria. However, certain individuals with sensitive intestines may experience severe indigestion as a result of consuming these foods, drastically diminishing their quality of life. As a result of fermentation byproducts, these individuals have persistent symptoms of gas, bloating, stomach discomfort, and distension. Insufficient or excessive absorption of water by the small intestine can result in constipation or diarrhoea, respectively.

Who might benefit from a low-FODMAP diet?

People diagnosed with irritable bowel syndrome (IBS) and small intestine bacterial overgrowth are frequently advised to follow a low-FODMAP diet for brief periods (SIBO). According to studies, the majority of individuals with these diseases benefit from diet. It can be used as a short-term elimination diet by anyone with digestive issues who wishes to identify the offending substances. An elimination diet entails eliminating common trigger foods and reintroducing them gradually to determine how your body reacts. The low-FODMAP diet is one of the many elimination diets you can use to identify food sensitivities.

2 .2 IRRITATED BOWEL DISEASE (IBS)

The syndrome known as irritable bowel syndrome affects the large intestine (IBS). Constipation, diarrhoea, bloating, gas, and cramps are among the symptoms and warning signs. IBS is a chronic disorder requiring long-term treatment.

Only a small percentage of IBS patients exhibit severe symptoms and signs. Some people can manage their symptoms by controlling their diet, lifestyle, and stress levels. Medication and psychotherapy may be utilised to treat severe symptoms.

IBS does not alter intestinal tissue or increase the risk of colorectal cancer.

Spastic colitis, irritable colon, mucous colitis, and irritable colon are alternative terms for IBS. It is unrelated to other gastrointestinal disorders and distinct from inflammatory bowel disease.

IBS is a collection of coexisting digestive symptoms. The severity and duration of symptoms vary between individuals.

Under certain conditions, IBS can be detrimental to the digestive system. However, that is uncommon.

Chapter 3: What Is Irritable Bowel Syndrome, What Causes It, And How Does It Affect Digestion?

One in seven people have Irritable Bowel Syndrome (IBS), a functional gastrointestinal disorder. It is estimated that 210 to 8 10 million people in the United States and 10 to 2 0% of the global population suffer from it.

A functional gut disorder is one in which the gut's function is disrupted but there are no visible signs of damage or disease in the digestive tract (this is why doctors in the past had a hard time diagnosing it). Rather, IBS is frequently diagnosed as a cluster of intestinal symptoms that frequently occur together.

Among the possible symptoms are (but are not limited to):

Bloating (the feeling of increased pressure in the abdomen) (the feeling of increased pressure in the abdomen)

Distention (the actual measurable change in the diameter of the abdomen) (the actual measurable change in the diameter of the abdomen)

Excessive gas

Abdominal pain and cramps, which are occasionally dull aches and occasionally stabbing pains.

Changes in bowel movements: The light-bulb and/or bowel movement

The relief of abdominal pain following a bowel movement.

Nausea

Fatigue

Mucus in the faeces

It is essential that you see a doctor who can diagnose your condition. By obtaining an accurate diagnosis, you can rule out other, more serious conditions, such as Coeliac Disease, Endometriosis, and Inflammatory Bowel Disease (IBD).

What causes my IBS symptoms?

Sadly, the precise cause of irritable bowel syndrome is unknown. Therefore, if you are performing the doctor's rounds in search of an answer, you may not find one. It is believed that there may be different causes for different individuals; I am aware that this is not helpful in any way. What the researchers do know is that IBS is more prevalent in women than in men and in those under the age of 10 0..so people like me and probably you, hurrah!

However, it is not the result of any physical damage to the GI tract or disease, which is reassuring. There are, however, a number of factors that appear to play a role and trigger IBS symptoms; some you may already be aware of, while others may pique your interest and warrant further investigation.

Gut Dysbiosis

Gut dysbiosis typically results from an imbalance of beneficial to harmful bacteria in the gut. This can be the result of a bacterial or viral infection, such as a severe case of light-bulb fever (gastroenteritis). Invasion of pathogenic bacteria into the gastrointestinal tract can result in a loss of microbial diversity and alterations to the gut flora. This imbalance may inhibit digestion and exacerbate IBS symptoms.

Dysbiosis can also be caused by the overuse of antibiotics by modern medicine to treat common conditions. In addition to destroying harmful bacteria, they eliminate beneficial bacteria that are essential for gut health. Diet can also cause dysbiosis, as we will discuss below.

The Modern Western Diet

Low in fibre, fruits, and vegetables (the good stuff), and high in processed foods, animal fat, saturated and hydrogenated fats, salt, sugar, preservatives, and additives, the modern Western diet is typically deficient in fibre, fruits, and vegetables (the not so good stuff). It has been demonstrated that this low-fiber, highly processed diet reduces the diversity of microbial species in the gut, alters the composition of bacterial communities, and weakens the gut lining.

This can have a negative impact on our gut microbiome because it creates the ideal breeding ground for an overgrowth of harmful bacteria, which can engulf and eradicate our healthy gut flora. This imbalance (gut dysbiosis) can lead to a variety of digestive disorders, such as irritable bowel syndrome (IBS), as very well as other conditions, including inflammatory bowel disease (IBD), type 2 diabetes, and depression.

A high-fiber, plant-based diet (rich in prebiotics) is ideal for repopulating the gut with healthy bacteria; it also aids in weight loss, blood sugar levels, and constipation. However, those of us with irritable bowel syndrome must proceed slowly. This is because many of us begin with a compromised digestive system. If we go all in, we can expect our IBS symptoms (excessive gas, stomach cramps, etc.) to become unbearable.

We must gradually increase our fibre consumption, thereby increasing the number of healthy bacteria in our gut and allowing us to consume larger high-fiber portions. More health benefits from larger portions = fewer IBS symptoms. But keep in mind that this must be done slowly.

The low Fodmap diet in conjunction with the Monash University App is beneficial because it specifies the portion sizes to consume initially to reduce digestive discomfort.

General Knowledge

Irritable bowel syndrome is a dysfunction of the digestive system. The condition is characterised by diarrhoea, abdominal cramps, and spasms. Psychological shocks and stress can result in deviance. IBS is most prevalent in women between the ages of 210 and 8 0, although it has been documented in children and adolescents.

This condition has no impact on the consistency or composition of faeces. The disease poses no threat to life and does not result in pathological alterations to the structure of the intestine; it only causes abdominal pain.

22

Irritable bowel syndrome is caused by the factors listed below:

Infectious pathologies (Crohn's disease, GERD, acute intestinal diseases), heredity, the effects of medications, and the acceleration or inhibition of intestinal motility

IBS is characterised by the occurrence of the following symptoms:

General malaise, abdominal pain, constipation or diarrhoea, the sensation of an incomplete bowel movement, bloating, increased gas formation, fatigue, anxiety, mucus in the stool, chills, and headache are all symptoms of irritable bowel syndrome (IBS).

Irritable bowel syndrome diet (IBS)

See a doctor immediately if you notice a change in the colour of your faeces or a sudden loss of weight.

Diet and IBS

Symptoms of IBS are frequently treated with dietary and lifestyle modifications. Understanding what is causing your IBS can help you determine the most effective treatment options. In some cases, medical and/or psychological treatment is advised.

Certain foods and behaviours, such as alcoholic and caffeinated beverages and smoking, are believed to trigger hives. If you are experiencing IBS symptoms, you should consult your doctor immediately. If no underlying health issues are identified, you may be referred to a nutritionist. A nutrition professional can help you understand what may be triggering your symptoms and guide you through any necessary lifestyle adjustments.

When it comes to diet and IBS, there is no "one size fits all" approach, so maintaining a food diary can be beneficial. The diet that works for one person may not work for you; therefore, knowing how you react to various foods can help you control your symptoms. If a particular food makes your stomach hurt, write it down. If a specific food appears to alleviate symptoms, include it in the lt.

Once you have compiled a list of recurrent trigger foods, you and your nutritionist can develop a diet plan for IBS that is specific to your symptoms.

Fibre

Fibre san rlau a big rart in managing symptoms of IBS. A professional may therefore recommend that you adjust the amount of fibre in your diet.

There are two types of cellulose, soluble and insoluble. Insoluble fibre cannot be digested by the body, whereas soluble fibre can (because it dissolves in water). If you suffer from constipation, drinking more water and increasing the amount of soluble fibre in your diet can help.

These foods contain soluble fibre:

rue barleu oats golden linseeds

root vegetables fruit

Foods sontaining insoluble fibre inslude:

Whole-grain bread with bran, nuts, and seeds.

Low FODMAP diet

If you experience frequent or persistent bloating, your nutritionist may recommend the low FODMAP diet, which is believed to be effective in managing IBS symptoms.

FODMAP is an acronym for fermentable oligofructose, disaccharides, monosaccharides, and oligosaccharides. These types of carbohydrates are difficult for the gut to absorb and digest, which means they ferment in the large intestine. The fermentation process causes the release of gases, resulting in painful bloating.

A low FODMAP diet involves limiting your consumption of certain high-FODMAP foods, such as certain fruits, vegetables, wheat germ, and dairy. If you are considering a low FODMAP diet, it is advised that you seek the assistance of a qualified professional. Without effort, the diet can be difficult to adhere to and, in some cases, can lead to digestive issues or nutritional deficiencies. A qualified dietitian can ensure that your diet is healthy and well-balanced while monitoring your symptoms and guiding you along the way.

Chapter 4: Diabetes tips: Controlling and Living With Diabetes

Controlling underlying conditions and maintaining nutrition

Controlling underlying conditions

High levels of glucose (sugar) in the blood tend to slow gastric emptying. Therefore, it is essential to reduce blood glucose levels in diabetic rats to near-normal levels through diet and medication. Individuals with a deficiency of thyroid hormone (hypothyroidism) should be treated with thyroid hormone. If there are bezoars, they must be eliminated (uuallu endosorsallu).

Maintaining nutrition

Patients with mild gastroparesis usually can be successfully managed with pain relievers and pro-motility medications, but patients with severe gastroparesis often require repeated hospitalizations to correct dehydration, and malnutrition, to control symptoms. Options for treating dehydration and malnutrition include:

Intravenous fluids to correct dehydration and replenish electrolytes if nutrition is adequate but symptoms occasionally interrupt the intake of even liquid food.

Enteral nutrition which provides liquid food directly into the small intestine, bypassing the paralyzed stomach.

Intravenous total parenteral nutrition (TPN) provides calories and nutrients (TPN is a fluid containing glucose, amino acids, lipids, minerals, and vitamins-everything that is needed for adequate nutrition-intravenously. The fluid usually is delivered into a large vein via a catheter in the arm or upper chest.)

Doctors generally recommend enteral nutrition over TPN because long-term TPN use is associated with catheter infection and liver damage. Infection can spread through the blood to the rest of the body, a serious condition called sepsis. Catheter-related sepsis often requires treatment with intravenous antibiotics and removal of the infected catheter or replacement with a new catheter. TPN can also cause liver damage, typically manifesting as abnormal liver tests in the blood. TPN-induced liver damage is typically mild and reversible (liver test abnormalities return to normal after cessation of TPN), but rare instances of irreversible liver failure have been reported. Sush liver failure mau require liver transplantation. Enteral nutrition is effective and safe. Common methods of administering enteral nutrition include nasojejunal tubes and jejunostomy tubes. The jejunum is the segment of the small intestine just beyond the duodenum, which is the first segment of the small intestine beyond the stomach. Both the nasojejunal tube and the jejunostomy tube are intended to bypass the stomach and deliver nutrients to the jejunum, where they can be absorbed. A naojejunal tube is a long, thin satheter inserted (typically by a radiologist or gastroenterologist) through the nasal cavity into the stomach. The tip of the nasojejunal tube was subsequently advanced from the stomach into the small intestine. Often this must be done during urrer GI endossoru. Liquid nutrients that can be delivered to the small intestine via the nasojejunal tube. Nasojejunal tubes are generally safe, but there are disadvantages and discomfort associated with having a tube in the nose. The most common problems associated with nasojejunal tubes are accidental or intentional removal of the ratent, clogging of the tube by solidified nutritional solutions, and arraton (backup of tomash sontent into the lungs, which can result in pneumonia).

A jejunotomu is a satheter that is positioned drestlu within the jejunum. It may be performed during standard abdominal surgery, using minimally invasive techniques (lararosoru), or by a radiologist with specialised training. With a jejunostomy, the surgeon makes an incision through the abdominal wall's skin and into the jejunum. Before a jejunostomy is inserted, a trial of nasojejunal nutrition is typically administered to ensure that the small bowel is not affected by the same motility disorder as the stomach and that nutritional liquids will be tolerated by the small intestine.

Chapter 5: What medication relieves nausea and vomiting from gastroparesis?

These include anti-nausea medications such as prochlorperazine and promethazine, serotonin antagonists such as ondansetron, and anticholinergic drugs.

Nonsteroidal ant-nflammatoru drug (NSAID) ush as ibuprofen (Motrin) and narroxen (Aleve), low doe trsusls antidepressants ush as amtrrtulne (Elavil, Ender), drug that blosk nerves that ene ran ush a gaba (Duragesic). (However, narsots as a group tend to increase sontraton and decrease emrtung of the tomash; therefore, they should be avoided or used with caution in patients with gastroparesis.

Elestrsal rasng of the tomash analogous to sardas pacing for the treatment of an abnormally slow heartbeat and involves the placement of a pacemaker.

Surgery: Surgery is often used to treat gastroparesis. The goal of surgery is to create a larger orenng between the stomach and the intestine to aid in the emptying of the stomach.

If gastroparesis is caused by a reversible condition, such as pancreatitis, the symptom will disappear when the underlying condition resolves. In some patients with diabetes, better control of their blood sugar will improve eructation.

If there is no exceptional sauce, gastroparesis is rarely cured. With time, it may become burdensome.

Gatrorare is extremely difficult to treat when there are assomranung motltu dorders of the small intestine's musle.

36

What's new with gatrorare?

The most recent experimental treatment for gastroparesis is botulinum toxin injection into the pylorus. The ruloru is the narrow passageway by which food travels from the stomach to the duodenum. Similar to the tomash, the ruloru is a musular organ. Most of the time, the ruloru slowed due to continual constriction of the pyloric muscle. Intermttentlu, it opens and allows esreton to enter the small entrance. After a meal, the ruloru is crucial for measuring the rate of stomach emptying. Although the musle of the tomash are always weak in gatrorare, the musle of the ruloru remains trong and sontrasted while the ruloru remains relatively sluggish. It was hypothesised that if the ruler's muscle was weakened, food would be expelled from the stomach more easily. Although the initial results were positive, subsequent research has

37

failed to confirm the efficacy of botulinum toxin. Although initial results with botulinum toxin were positive, subsequent research has not confirmed the benefit. Its use should be considered extraordinary. Although a surgical procedure known as rulororlatu has been used in the past to treat problems with emphysema of the throat, it is a major operation with mixed results regarding its efficacy.

The Medieval Definition of Gatrorare

Gatrorare: A disease of the stomach lining or the nerves controlling the lining that causes the lining to stop working. Gatrorare results in inadequate food grinding by the stomach and poor food passage from the stomach into the intestine. Gatrorare may be associated with small intestinal and colonic raralu. The most prevalent underlying condition is diabetes mellitus. Gatrorare is diagnosed through a gastric emptying study. Typically, it is treated with medications that stimulate the stomach mucus to contract.

Chess for the Heart Deae

The leading cause of death and illness among diabetics is cardiovascular disease, also known as heart disease. One study found that over 810 percent of diabetic rats also have high blood pressure, a predictor of heart disease. If you have hurertenon, like the majority of diabetics, it is crucial that you check your blood sugar regularly at home. Here are some techniques for performing the sorrestlu:

Choose a home blood pressure monitor that encircles your arm. These take reading more slowly to the heart and are deemed more reliable as a result.

If you do not wish to manually inflate and measure your blood pressure, choose an automated monitor. Accurate models are available for less than thirty dollars and are covered by insurance.

Several times per week, measure your blood pressure twice in the morning and once at night. Relax as you complete the task; anxiety can increase blood pressure.

Choose a time at least thirty minutes after exercising and consuming caffeine, alcohol, or tobacco. This may disrupt your reading.

Place both feet comfortably on the ground. Rest your chair against your sofa. Place your arm on a table-like surface. Wait five minutes before beginning your reading.

Remember these numbers: a normal blood pressure reading is 2 20/80. Prehurertension is sonsidered 2 20-2 6 9/80-89. Above 2 8 0/90, blood pressure is considered to be high.

Take notes on your reading. Write them down or record them on your smartphone, and bring them to your professor on your next visit. Your physician can prescribe a blood pressure-lowering drug and start you on a medication that can help you better manage your hypertension.

Bandage Up

Individuals with diabetes have a decreased sell growth response to wounds. This is one reason why you are more susceptible to foot ulcers, a leading cause of hospitalisation in this population. The American Diabetes Association suggests treating sut with clean bandages immediately. Major burns, cuts, and infections are serious enough for diabetics to require immediate treatment. On a number of fronts, including tissue engineering and stem cell research, scientists are working to find a solution to this serious health issue.

Extinguish the Smoke

Everyone knows that smoking is unhealthy. However, this is absolutely true for people with diabetes. Doctors have known for a long time that diabetic smokers are more likely to develop heart disease, kidney disease, high blood pressure, vision problems, and nerve damage. Now you believe you know what. A shemtru professor examined human blood amrle and discovered something strange. Simply adding nicotine to blood samples reduces blood glucose levels. As it turns out, nicotine (present in nicotine gum and patches in addition to cigarettes) increases the risk of developing diabetes by 6 0% to 8 0%. And if you already have diabetes, nicotine makes it more difficult to manage your symptoms. Nicotine is notoriously addictive, and withdrawal can be difficult. Your shanse are improved if you request helr. Tell your doctor that you want to quit smoking and ask for advice and resources to help you on your journey to a healthier you.

Chapter 6: How To Follow A Diet Low In Fodmap

A low-FODMAP diet consists of three stages and is more complicated than you might think.

Stage 2 : Limitations

This phase requires the avoidance of all foods high in FODMAPs. Read this article if you're uncertain which foods are high in FODMAPs. People who follow this diet frequently believe they must avoid all FODMAPs indefinitely, despite the fact that this phase should only last between 6 and 8 weeks. This is because the inclusion of FODMAPs in the diet is essential for gut health. While some individuals experience a reduction in symptoms within the first week, others must wait the full eight weeks. Once you've obtained sufficient relief from your digestive symptoms, you can proceed to the next phase. Refer to the What If Your Symptoms Don't Improve section if your stomach symptoms have not improved after eight weeks. The following.

Reintroduction constitutes Phase 2

This phase involves reintroducing high-FODMAP foods systematically.

The objectives are twofold:

Determine which FODMAPs you can tolerate. Few individuals are sensitive to them all.

Determine the amount of FODMAPs you can tolerate. This is known as one's "threshold level."

In this step, you sample individual foods for three days each.

45

It is recommended that you complete this step alongside a qualified dietitian who can guide you through the proper foods. Alternatively, this application can assist you in deciding which foods to reintroduce. It is essential to remember that a low-FODMAP diet must be maintained throughout this stage. This means that even if you are able to tolerate certain high-FODMAP foods, you must continue to limit them until Stage 6 . In contrast to the majority of individuals with food allergies, individuals with IBS may be able to tolerate small amounts of FODMAPs.

Even though digestive symptoms can be debilitating, they do not cause long-term harm to the body.

Stage 6 : Personalization

This phase is also known as the "modified low-FODMAP diet," which means that you continue to restrict some

FODMAPs. The quantity and type, however, are tailored to your individual tolerance, as determined in Stage 2. To increase the variety and adaptability of the diet, it is essential to reach this final level. These characteristics are associated with improved compatibility over the long term, life quality, and intestinal health.

Three Things To Do Prior To Starting

There are three steps to take before beginning a diet.

Confirm That You Have IBS

There are numerous causes of digestive symptoms, some of which are harmful and others more severe. Unfortunately, there is no diagnostic test that conclusively confirms IBS. In order to rule out more serious conditions, such as celiac disease, inflammatory bowel disease, and colorectal cancer, it is recommended that you first see a doctor. Once these conditions have been ruled out, your physician can confirm your IBS using the formal diagnostic criteria for IBS. To be diagnosed with IBS, all three criteria must be met.

• Frequent stomach pain: at least one day per week on average during the past three months.

•Stool symptom: Two or more of the following must be true: associated with defecation, associated with a change in stool frequency, or associated with a change in stool distribution.

• Persistent symptoms: meeting criteria for the last three months, with symptoms present for at least eight months prior to diagnosis.

First-Line Diet Strategies

The low-FODMAP diet requires considerable time and resources. This is why, in clinical practise, it is considered second-line dietary advice and is only used in a subset of IBS patients who do not respond to first-line strategies. Here you can find additional information about first-line nutritional advice.

Plan Forward

If you are not prepared, you may find it difficult to adhere to the schedule. Here are some tirs:

• Determine what to purchase: Ensure you have access to a credible low-FODMAP food list. Below is a list of locations where you can find them.

• Remove all high-FODMAP foods from your refrigerator and pantry.

Create a low-FODMAP shopping list before heading to the grocery store so you know which foods to purchase and which to avoid.

• Read menus beforehand: Familiarize yourself with low-FODMAP menu options so that you are prepared when dining out.

How long must I follow a low FODMAP diet?

The low FODMAP diet has three phases: elimination, reintroduction, and individualization.

Phase of elimination - All FODMAP-rich foods should be eliminated. This phase typically lasts two weeks, but may last longer if you experience more severe gastro-intestinal distress. The general recommendation is to adhere to this phase of the diet until you no longer experience IBS-related symptoms, which varies by individual.

This phase typically begins around week three and lasts for four to six weeks. One food at a time is reintroduced into the diet in small quantities and then gradually increased. If there are no accompanying digestive problems, the food is reintroduced. You would continue eliminating FODMAP-containing foods one by one until you were able to identify the specific foods that exacerbated your IBS symptoms.

Individualization: Once a list of acceptable foods and foods that trigger IBS symptoms has been compiled, a meal plan should be developed. Your diet should be well-balanced and comprise a variety of food groups and nutrients. The amount of food that an individual with IBS can tolerate varies considerably. You might be able to tolerate the vast majority of FODMAP-containing foods, none at all, or any amount. Only by attempting it will you discover the solution! Your personalised meal plan will help you manage your IBS symptoms if you adhere to it.

Remember that the objective is not to eliminate all FODMAPS. The healthiest foods are those that are low in FODMAPS. Sometimes, eliminating foods high in FODMAPs can lead to deficiencies in fibre, protein, and vitamins A, C, and D. Because of this, we recommend working with a registered dietitian or nutritionist if you decide to use a low FODMAP diet to treat IBS.

FIRST PART

What are considered FODMAPs?

FODMAP stands for fermentable oligo-, di-, and monosaccharides and polyols.

Even if they cannot be digested, these short-chain carbohydrates are osmotically active, meaning they push water into the digestive tract.

In addition, because they cannot be digested, they are fermented by your gut bacteria, resulting in an increase in gas and short-chain fatty acids.

Consequently, FODMAPs are well-known for causing digestive system symptoms such as gas, bloating, stomach pain, and altered bowel habits ranging from constipation to diarrhoea or a combination of the two.

In fact, more than sixty percent of IBS patients claim that these carbohydrates either cause or exacerbate their symptoms.

A wide variety of foods contain varying amounts of FODMAPs. Some foods contain a variety of them, while others contain only one. The four major dietary sources of FODMAPs are:

Nuts, beans, artichokes, garlic, and onion; wheat, rye, and oligosaccharides.

Lactose is a disaccharide found in milk, yoghurt, soft cheese, ice cream, buttermilk, condensed milk, and whipped cream.

Apples, pears, watermelons, and mangoes are high in fructose, as are honey, agave nectar, and high fructose corn syrup.

Polyols; The low-calorie sweeteners xylitol and isomalt, which are found in sugar-free gum and mints, as very well as mannitol and sorbitol, which are found in apples, pears, cauliflower, stone fruits, mushrooms, and snow peas.

What foods are permitted on the low-FODMAP diet?

The average daily consumption of FODMAPs from a low- or high-FODMAP diet is 0.10 2 ounces (2 10 6 0 grammes).

A low FODMAP diet, on the other hand, aims to limit your consumption to 0.02 ounces (0.10 grammes) per sitting, which corresponds to 0.080.2 ounces (2.10 6 grammes) if you adhere to the recommendation to consume small, frequent meals.

Thankfully, many foods have naturally low FODMAP levels. Here is a list of foods that adhere to the low-FODMAP diet.

Beef, chicken, fresh eggs , fish, lamb, pig, prawns, tempeh, and tofu are examples of proteins.

Whole grains and complex carbohydrates include brown and white rice, lentils, cassava, potatoes, quinoa, corn, and oats.

Strawberries, blueberries, raspberries, honeydew melon, grapes, limes, guava, starfruit, cantaloupe, and pineapple are some examples of fruits.

Cucumber, pumpkin, bell peppers, radishes, bok choy, carrots, celery, eggplant, kale, tomatoes, and zucchini are examples of vegetables.

Almonds (ten per session maximum), macadamia nuts, pecans, peanuts, walnuts, and pine nuts.

Seeds such as Pumpkin seeds, sesame seeds, sunflowers, and linseed seeds.

Lactose-free milk, Greek yoghurt, Parmesan, Colby, cheddar, and mozzarella cheeses are dairy products.

Coconut and extra virgin olive oils are examples of oils.

The following beverages are available: water and peppermint tea

Cumin, saffron, cinnamon, paprika, coriander, cardamom, certain chile-based ingredients, ginger, mustard, pepper, salt, white rice vinegar, and wasabi powder are condiments.

Even though black tea, green tea, and coffee are low in FODMAPs, it is generally not recommended to include them in a low FODMAP diet because they can exacerbate IBS symptoms.

Additionally, it is essential to examine ingredient lists of packaged foods for additional FODMAPs. Food manufacturers may use FODMAPs for a variety of purposes, including as prebiotics, fat substitutes, and low-calorie sugar substitutes.

Chapter 7: Vegan summer squash soup with a low fod map

Our Vegan Low FODMAP Summer Suah Sour with Cosonut is made with no FODMAP rattu ran uah (alo relled "pattypan"), sosonut milk, and rse like turmers and coriander. Yukon gold rotatoe add body, flavour, and boost the solor, along with no FODMAP sarrot.

The inspiration for our resres comes from a variety of places.

You mght not be famlar wth patty ran uah. It is the yellow round one in the image below.

Therefore, this recipe for Vegan Low FODMAP Summer Squash Soup is a trifecta featuring No FODMAP carrots, potatoes, and patty pan squash.

Not every summer suah is identical.

Yellow summer squash have not been tested for FODMAPs, but zucchini has been, and it has a significantly different FODMAP content than pumpkin.

You could easy make this dish with yellow squash, but we do not recommend doing so until you are comfortable with your IBS symptoms and have passed the Challenge Phase.

Vegetable Stock Low in FODMAPs

For this soup, you will need Low FODMAP Vegetable Broth. We offer a homemade version, but there are also commercially prepared broths that you may use.

Whatever Low FODMAP Vegetable Broth you use, its flavour will have a significant impact on the final product (and any soup it enhances, for that matter). Every homemade batch will be different, and each brand will have a unique flavour.

You can adjust the flavour of this dish by adding more or less of the rosemary. The rattu pan uah and potatoes, which easy make up the majority of the our, are extremely mild and will be brought to life by the broth of your choice and your seasoning.

Flourless Chocolate Olive Oil Cake

Chocolate cake Serves: 2 2 Prep: 2 10 minutes Cook: 10 10 minutes

As dietitians, many people think we have a perfect diet, full of fruit and vegetables and that we don't go near desserts or sweets, but that couldn't be further from the truth! Like most people, we love our desserts and we want to promote balance, so the occasional slice of cake is more than ok with us.

ingredients

- regular olive oil 2 10 0 g
- 1 cup good quality cocoa powder, sifted 10 0 g
- 1 cup boiling water 2 210 g
- 2 Tsp vanilla extract 2 0 g
- 2 ¼ cup almond meal/flour (for a nut free option use 2 210 g/8 .8 oz plain, premade gluten free flour) 2 10 0 g
- 1 Tsp bicarbonate soda 2 g
- 2 pinch salt 2 g

- caster sugar 200 g
- 6 large fresh eggs fresh eggs
- **raspberries or strawberries to serve**

Method

1. Preheat your oven to 2 70°C/6 6 8°F. Grease a 26 cm spring-form tin with a little oil and line with baking paper

2. Add the sifted cocoa powder to a jug and which in the boiling water, stirring until you have a smooth but still a little runny paste. Whisk in vanilla extract and set aside.

3. In another small bowl, combine the ground almonds (or flour) with the bicarb soda and the salt.

4. Place the sugar, olive oil and fresh eggs fresh eggs into the bowl of a freestanding mixer with the paddle attachment (or a regular bowl and whisk of your choice) and beat well for about 6

minutes until you have a pale, aerated and thick creamy mixture.

5. Turn the speed down and pour in the cocoa mixture, whisking as you go, when fully combined, add the almond meal (or flour) and combine.

6. Pour the batter into the prepared tin and bake for 8 0-8 10 minutes. The sides should be set but the top will look damp and a little soft. Nigella's tip is a cake skewer should come out mainly clean with a few sticky crumbs clinging to it.

7. Let the cake cool in the tin on a wire rack for 2 0 minutes before serving.

Eggplant-Kale Caponata Lasagna

- Prep Time 2 0 minutes
- Easy easy cook Time 10 0 minutes
- Total Time 2 hour
- Servings 6

Ingredients

- 2 tablespoons olive oil
- 2 medium eggplant 6 /8 pound, diced
- 1 teaspoon sea salt
- 1 teaspoon red chili flakes
- 2 medium vine or Roma tomato diced
- 8 ounces frozen chopped kale or 2 bunch finely chopped
- 2 cups low FODMAP tomato sauce 2 6 ounces
- 2 tablespoons golden raisins
- 2 tablespoon balsamic vinegar
- ¼ cup torn basil leaves divided
- 9 ounces gluten-free no boil lasagna noodles about 6 sheets
- 8 ounces plant-based ricotta optional

• 10 ounces shredded mozzarella I used a combo of part-skim and fresh mozz

Instructions

• Preheat the oven to 6 10 0 degrees.

• In a large skillet, heat the olive oil. Sauté the eggplant over medium-high heat until beginning to soften, about 8 minutes. Add the salt and red pepper flakes. Stir in the tomatoes, scrapping up any brown bits from the bottom of the pan. Sauté until the tomatoes have softened, about 6 minutes. Add the kale and continue to sauté until very wilted and the liquid has evaporated, about 8 minutes more.

• Remove from the heat and add the raisins, balsamic and half the basil.

• Spread 1 cup of the tomato sauce in the bottom of a 9 x 2 6 casserole dish. Arrange your first layer of noodles on top, making sure they overlap slightly. Slather the noodles with half the ricotta, if using, followed by half the eggplant mixture, followed by another 1 cup sauce and ¼ cup mozzarella. Repeat the layers once more.

• Finish the lasagna with a final layer of noodles, tomato sauce, the remaining cheese and basil leaves.

• Bake in the oven for 6 0-8 0 minutes, or until the noodles are tender and the top of the lasagna is beginning to brown.

• Allow the lasagna to rest for 10 minutes before cutting it into slabs and serving.

Stuffed Sweet Potatoes

You cannot really go wrong with stuffed potatoes, correct? It always hits the mark, and the sudden storm is going to actually bring this dish to life. The shskrea are dunked in an aromatic sauce and sprinkled with soy sauce before being tossed with baked potatoes. Curru Chskrea Stuffed Sweet Potatoes - A stale and flavourless dish. Chskrea was steeped in a fragrant coconut ause. The finest vegan comfort food!

Ingredients

- 2 cup or more broth or water

- 2 cup coconut milk replace with broth or water

- 2 teaspoon cayenne pepper optional

- 4 green onions chopped

- 1-5 cups fresh leaf spinach

- 4 tablespoons or more chopped parsley

- Salt to taste
- 1/2 cup canola oil
- 5-10 tablespoon curry powder
- 2 large onion diced

- 4 teaspoons minced garlic

- 2 - teaspoon ground allspice

- 2 - teaspoon ground nutmeg spice

- 3 teaspoon smoked paprika

- 4 teaspoons fresh or dried thyme

- 2 - teaspoon cumin spice

- 2 - teaspoon white pepper.

- 4 cans of chickpeas drained

- 1-5 cups of cubed potatoes

- 1 1   - tablespoon bouillon chicken powder optional

Instructions

1. Heat up large sauce-pan with oil, and add onions, garlic, thyme, cumin spice, all spice, smoked paprika, nutmeg and curry powder, stir occasionally for about 5-10 minutes until onions is translucent.

2. Then add potatoes, stir and sauté for about 5-10 more minutes.

3. Add coconut milk /stock / water if necessary to prevent any burns

4. Next add chickpeas, green onion and broth.

5. Bring to a boil and let it simmer until sauce thickens, it might take about 5-10 minutes.

6. Lastly throw in some spinach ,parsley, adjust for salt, pepper and stew consistency.

7. Stir for about a minute until spinach is wilted .Serve warm

8. While curry is simmering.

9. Easy easy cook sweet potatoes in your microwave: Prick the potatoes all over with a fork.

10. Microwave on high for 5-10 minutes or until sweet potatoes is tender, turning the potatoes once.

11. Clean and dry the sweet potatoes, poke holes into the sweet potatoes, place in the microwave and easy easy cook for about 8 minutes.

12. Remove, let easy easy cook for a couple of minutes Slice open the sweet potatoes and stuff! If your sweet potatoes are large, cut them in half.

Low Fodmap Carrot Consommé

INGREDIENTS:

- 10 black peppercorns
- 4 whole cloves
- 4 bay leaves
- 4 sprigs fresh thyme
- 2 celery stalk, trimmed and cut into large chunks
- Kosher salt
- 6 quarts (2.8 L) water
- 8 - pounds (2 .8 kg) carrots, trimmed, peeled and cut into large chunks
- 2 cup (72 g) chopped leeks, green parts only
- 2- inches (10 cm) fresh ginger, peeled and cut in half lengthwise

PREPARATION:

1. Combine all of the ingredients in a large stockpot, cover, bring to a boil over high heat, then adjust heat and simmer for 4 hours.
2. Remove from heat, cool briefly, then carefully pour through a cheesecloth lined fine-mesh strainer into another large pot.
3. Discard vegetables. Taste the consommé and season with salt as desired.
4. Re-heat and serve.
5. Consommé can also be cooled and refrigerated in an airtight conatiner for up to 6 days.
6. Reheat on stovetop.

Peanut Butter And And Vanana Night-Time Oats

INGREDIENTS:

- 8 tbsp. peanut butter, natural and no sugar added
- 4 cups almond milk, unsweetened
- 2 Tsp. ground cinnamon
- 4 cups gluten-free rolled oats
- 8 Tsp. chia seeds
- 4 medium bananas, mashed

DIRECTIONS:

1. Blend cinnamon, almond milk, peanut butter, bananas, chia seeds, and oats in a glass dish.
2. Toss to combine fully and cover with a layer of plastic wrap.
3. Transfer to the refrigerator and serve the next morning immediately if you desire it cold. If you prefer hot, nuke in the microwave for 90 seconds before enjoying.

Banana Nut Quinoa Muffins

Ingredients

Dry Ingredients:

8 tsp. baking powder

4 tsp. baking soda

2 tsp. salt

1-5C quinoa flour

2 C quinoa flakes

1 C walnuts or pecans, chopped

2 Tbsp. cinnamon

Wet Ingredients:

8 very ripe bananas, mashed

8 flax fresh eggs (or 8 real fresh eggs)

1/2   C maple syrup

1 cup almond milk

Directions

1. Preheat your oven to 6 10 0 degrees F.
2. First, prepare your flax fresh eggs and place them in the
3. fridge to gel.
4. Then, in a large bowl, mix all dry ingredients. In a
5. separate smaller bowl, mix mashed bananas, almondmilk, and maple syrup, then mix in gelled flax fresh eggs .
6. Add wet ingredients to dry ingredients and stir until more or less uniform.

7. Spoon batter into greased muffin pans; place in the oven for 20 minutes. Fork check to test the

8. done-ness.

!

Chapter 8: How Does One Commence A Low-Fodmap Diet?

The low-FODMAP diet consists of three foods. Shah advises relying on a registered dietitian for guidance on an elimination diet because the foods that are eliminated are not clearly identified. Below the rrotosol that he administers to patients at the clinics:

Phase 2 : Elimination

Set an expiration date and eliminate all high-FODMAP foods from the diet. In this situation, it is essential to have a registered dietitian on your team, as they can provide guidance on proper food preparation. "In order to be successful, it is necessary to understand how to eliminate FODMAPs in different life scenarios at work, while travelling, and at home, as very well as how to find alternatives in each setting," says Shah.

Extra credit for planning ahead and replacing high-FODMAP foods with low-FODMAP alternatives. The delay is between two and four weeks.

Phase 2 consists of reintroduction

Shah explains that the primary objective of phase 2 is to identify your food triggers. While there is no definitive way to reintroduce food, the common recommendation is to reintroduce one FODMAP at a time with a small amount of food. Therefore, reintroducing lastoe may involve drinking one glass of sow's milk and observing how your body reacts. Reintroducing frustose may require half a watermelon.

During this time, you will continue to follow a low-FODMAP diet in order to determine which foods trigger your symptoms. Keep a food journal on hand, using either an app on your smartphone or an old-fashioned notebook, to record your umrtom. This rhae lasts between six and eight weeks.

Phase 6 : Individualization

"We continue to expand the low-FODMAP diet by consuming well-tolerated FODMAPs and eliminating those that are problematic," says Shah. She notes that t' unlkelu anu one food must be avoided entirely. Generally, bothersome foods should not be consumed daily or in large quantities, as tolerance is frequently dose-dependent.

Keep in mind that you do not have to be perfect throughout the entire process. "The objective is not to have a FODMAP-free diet, but to reduce FODMAPs in the diet in order to modify GI symptoms," explains Scarlata. "Added stress with diet changes can exacerbate gut symptoms, which is not the objective here," she said.

The advantages of a low FODMAP diet

A low FODMAP diet excludes foods high in FODMAPs. Ssentfs evidence suggests that people with IBS may benefit from this eating pattern.

• May alleviate digestive symptoms IBS symptoms include abdominal pain, bloating, reflux, flatulence, and bowel urgency. Needle to au, these symptoms may be incapacitating. A low FODMAP diet has been demonstrated to reduce both stomach pain and bloating. Evidence from four high-quality studies suggests that a low FODMAP diet increases the likelihood of relief from stomach ache and bloating by 82 % and 710 %, respectively. Several additional studies indicate and imply that this diet also aids in the management of flatulence, diarrhoea, and constipation. A low FODMAP diet is now considered fast-line during fasting. Detaru theraru for IBS in numerous regions of the world.

• Mau improve your quality of life Individuals with irritable bowel syndrome frequently report a diminished quality of life due to severe digestive symptoms. This condition may impact social interactions and even workplace reformanse. Multiple studies indicate that a low FODMAP diet improves quality of life by significantly reducing gastrointestinal symptoms. Some evidence suggests that a diet that improves digestive symptoms may also reduce fatigue, depression, and anxiety while boosting energy and vitality.

Who must adhere to a low FODMAP diet?

A diet low in FODMAPs is not for everyone. Unless you have been diagnosed with IBS, this diet may be counterproductive. This is because most FODMAPs are fermentable, meaning they inhibit the growth of beneficial gut bacteria. Therefore, eliminating them could harm your intestinal bacteria, which could negatively impact your health. In addition, excluding several fruits and vegetables from your diet may result in vitamin and mineral deficiencies as very well as a significant reduction in your fibre intake, which may exacerbate constipation. Therefore, to ensure nutritional sufficiency and avoid potential complications, you should only follow the diet under the supervision of a dietitian with expertise in digestive disorders. If uou have IBS, consider this diet if you:

• have persistent gastrointestinal symptoms

• haven't resronded to stress management tratege • haven't responded to first-line dietary advice, such as adjusting meal size and frequency and reducing your intake of alcohol, caffeine, and other common trigger foods.

While there is some evidence that the diet may benefit other conditions, including diabetes and exercise-induced digestive issues, additional research is required. Due to the complexity of this diet, you should not try it for the first time while travelling or during a stressful period.

How to follow a FODMAP-restricted diet

A low FODMAP diet is complex and consists of three phases: • Phase 2 : Restriction

This phase requires strict avoidance of all foods high in FODMAPs. People who follow the diet often believe they must avoid all FODMAPs indefinitely, but this stage should only last 8 –8 weeks. This is because FODMAPs are so essential for gut health. Some patients experience improvement in symptoms within the first week, while others require the full eight weeks. Seventy-five to seventy-five percent of those who followed the diet plan experienced improvement in symptoms within six weeks. Once you have obtained sufficient relief from your digestive symptoms, you can proceed to the next stage.

• Stage 2: Reintrodustion

This stage involves the systematic reintroduction of high FODMAP foods. Although its duration varies by region, t tursallu lasts between 6 and 2 0 weeks.

The objectives of this phase are twofold:

• To determine which types of FODMAPs you can tolerate, as few people are sensitive to all of them, you must determine which types you can tolerate.

• to determine the amount of FODMAPs that you can tolerate, also called your "threshold level" In this step, you test small quantities of pet food for three days.

To avoid additive or sroover effects, it is recommended to remain on a strict low FODMAP diet while testing each food and wait 2–6 days before reintroducing a new food. Once you've established your baseline tolerance, you can assess your tolerance to higher doses, increased frequency of consumption, and combinations of high FODMAP foods; however, you should take a 2–6 day break between each test. It is best to take this step with the assistance of a registered dietitian who can guide you through the appropriate foods. It's also important to remember that, unlike individuals with most food allergies, who must completely avoid certain allergens, individuals with IBS can tolerate small amounts of FODMAP.

• Stage 6 : Personalization

This phase is also known as the "modified low FODMAP diet" because you continue to restrict some FODMAPs but reintroduce those that are very well tolerated. In other words, during this stage, the quantity and type of FODMAPs are tailored to your individual tolerance level, as determined in stage 2. The low FODMAP diet is neither a one-size-fits-all solution nor a long-term regimen. The ultimate goal is to reintroduce high FODMAP foods at a level of tolerance that you can tolerate. It is essential to proceed to the final stage in order to increase diet variety and flexibility. These characteristics are associated with improved long-term sleep, quality of life, and gut health.

There are three things to do before you begin.

Follow these three steps prior to beginning a low FODMAP diet.

• Verify that you have IBS digestive symptoms in a variety of forms, some harmless and others more severe. IBS symptoms are also common in a variety of other chronic conditions, including celiac disease, inflammatory bowel disease, defecation disorders, and multiple sclerosis. Therefore, you should consult a physician to rule out these other possibilities. Your doctor can confirm that you have IBS using the official IBS diagnostic criteria once these causes have been ruled out. To be diagnosed with IBS, you must satisfy all three of the following criteria. Chronic abdominal pain. In the past three months, our ran has occurred at least one day per week on average. The stool umrtom. Thee hould match two or more of the following: associated with defecation, associated with a change in stool frequency, or associated with an alteration in stool appearance. Persistent sumrtoms. You have experienced consistent symptoms for the past three months, with symptoms beginning at least six months prior to diagnosis.

• Tru lifestyle and dietaru modification strategies

The low FODMAP diet is a time- and resource-consuming endeavour. In some countries, this is considered second-line dietary advice and is only used for patients with IBS who do not respond to first-line strategies.

• Prepare ahead

It may be difficult to adhere to the low FODMAP diet's restrictions. Here are some tips to assist you in preparing: Determine what to buy. Ensure you have access to a sufficient supply of low FODMAP foods. Get rid of FODMAP-rich foods. Empty your refrigerator and pantry of food to prevent mistakes. Create a horrifying lt. Create a low

FODMAP shopping list before going to the supermarket so you know which foods to buy and which to avoid. Read menus in advanse. Be familiar with low FODMAP menu options so that you are prepared when dining out.

Chapter 9: Ibd - Treatment And Aetiology

Several variables may contribute to the improvement of IBD. For example, this may occur if the safe framework has an unpredictable reaction to microorganisms, pathogens, or food particles. This may provoke an inflammatory response in the stomach.

IBD is the result of a compromised immune system, although the precise cause of IBD is unknown. Potential causes are:

The immune system responds incorrectly to natural stimuli, such as an infection or microorganisms, resulting in irritation of the gastrointestinal tract.

There also has the appearance of being an inherited trait. Those with a family history of inflammatory bowel disease are likely to develop this inappropriate immune response.

IBD can cause several serious digestive tract complications, including:

Abundant digestive drainage from the ulcers' hole or internal rupture

As in Crohn's Fistulae (unusual entries) and perianal disease, a disease of the tissue surrounding the buttocks, this condition is limiting and impedes digestion. These conditions are more typical of Crohn's disease than ulcerative colitis.

Poisonous megacolon, which is an extreme expansion of the colon, undermines the veracity. This is more related to ulcerative colitis than Crohn's disease.

Lack of nutritious food

IBD MEDICATION

These diseases have become major medical concerns. With the introduction of designated biologic treatments, the improvement of more established treatments, such as immunomodulators and 10 -aminosalicylic acid, and a better understanding of the mucosal resistant framework and hereditary characteristics associated with the pathogenesis of IBD, the clinical treatment for inflammatory bowel disease (IBD) has advanced significantly in recent years. The purpose of IBD treatment is to induce and sustain remission. The ebb and flow treatment philosophy entails a move-forward strategy, transitioning to forceful, strong treatments when milder treatments with fewer potential side effects fail or when patients report a severe infection. This audit focuses on the distribution of medications for incendiary entrail infection.

The objective of treatment for fiery internal infections is to achieve abatement so that side effects disappear and to maintain reduction so that eruptions do not occur, while maximising patient satisfaction. The lining of the gastrointestinal tract recovers as a result of a decrease.

Potato & Egg Salad

Ingredients:

- 6 tbsp green onions/scallions (green tips only)
- 170 ml (2 /6 cup) mayonnaise
- 2 tbsp fresh lemon juice
- 2 tbsp wholegrain mustard
- Season with dark pepper
- 1600 g potato
- 250 g green beans
- 8 huge egg
- 2 red chili peppers
- 2 little cucumber
- 6 tbsp new chives

fresh lemon

Directions:

1. Scour and cut the potatoes into reduced down pieces (strip if vital).

2. Set up the green beans by cutting into little pieces.

3. Spot the potatoes in an enormous pan and cover with water.

4. Spot the cover on the pot and carry the water to a turning bubble over medium-high warmth.

5. At that point turn down the heat to medium-low and permit to bubble for 35 to 40 minutes until the potatoes are delicate.

6. Add the green beans to the pot, around 6 minutes before you channel the potatoes.

7. Enable the green beans to easy cook for 2 to 6 minutes, until delicate and brilliantly shaded.

8. Deplete and spot to the other side to cool.

9. While the potatoes cook, hard-heat up the fresh eggs . Spot the fresh eggs fresh eggs in a little pot of water and spread with cold water.

10.   Spot the pan over medium-high warmth and carry the water to a moving bubble.

11.   Permit to bubble for two minutes before turning the heat down to the least warmth setting.

12.   Easy cook for 1-5   minutes. Deplete and run the fresh eggs fresh eggs under cold water before stripping. Cut the fresh eggs fresh eggs into quarters.

13.   While the fresh eggs fresh eggs cook, set up the cucumber and red chili peppers. Strip the cucumber and cut into off sticks.

14. Deseed and bones the red ringer peppers. Finely hack the green onions/scallions and chives.

15. Easy make the plate of mixed greens dressing by combining the wholegrain mustard, mayonnaise, fresh lemon juice and two or three toils of dark pepper.

16. In an enormous bowl delicately combine the potatoes, green beans, hard-bubbled fresh eggs , cucumber, red chime peppers, green onions/scallions chives and plate of mixed greens dressing.

17. Season with a few drudgeries of dark pepper.

18. Enjoy yourself

Mediterranean Salad

Where peppers and chilies should be included in a low-FODMAP diet's list of recommended foods is the subject of considerable debate. Some listings lack them, while others contain them. It is acceptable to omit the peppers from this dish because they are not used in significant amounts. You won't be able to ignore the salad's extravagant flavours and hues.

- 2 teaspoon minced fresh oregano

- 1 teaspoon red pepper flakes (optional)

- 1 cup olive oil

- 4 tablespoons fresh fresh lemon juice

- 2 teaspoon minced fresh mint

Kosher Salt And Freshly Ground Black Pepper

- 1 roasted red bell pepper, peeled and cut into strips (about ¼ cup)

- 4 teaspoons brine-packed capers, rinsed

- 4 teaspoons pine nuts

- 4 ounces cubed aged Provolone cheese

- 4 ounces cubed salami

- 8 cups chopped romaine lettuce

- 4 fresh tomatoes, cut into wedges

- 1 1 cucumber, cut into thin slices

- 20 kalamata olives, pitted

- 8 anchovy fillets (optional)

2 .To easy make the dressing, in a small bowl, combine the olive oil, fresh lemon

juice, mint, oregano, and red pepper flakes and season with salt and pepper. Set aside.

2.In a large salad bowl, combine the romaine, tomatoes, cucumber, olives, anchovies bell pepper, capers, pine nuts, Provolone, and salami.

Add the dressing and toss until evenly coated.

6 .Serve immediately.

Minestrone

INGREDIENTS

- 2 Zucchini - cubed
- 2 Leek - finely chopped
- 20 Cherry Tomatoes
- 2 cup Frozen Peas
- 2 .10 litres of Water (or vegetable stock)
- 2 cube Vegetable Bouillon
- a handful of Rice Vermicelli (or other small pasta shapes)
- Salt and freshly ground Black Pepper
- A few fresh Basil Leaves, finely chopped
- Optional Topping: Grated Parmesan
-     10 tablespoons Extra Virgin Olive Oil
-     2 White Onion - finely chopped
-     2 clove Garlic - finely chopped
-     4 Potatoes - peeled and cubed (or sweet potatoes)
-     400g Pumpkin - peeled and cubed
-     4 Carrots - thickly sliced
-     2 Celery Stalk - thickly sliced

- 2 small Broccoli head - cut into small pieces

Preparation

1. Heat the extra virgin olive oil in a large pot on low fire, add the onion and garlic, and saute for 5-10 minutes until the onion is translucent.
2. Add all the vegetables, the hard vegetables first, followed by softer ones, except the frozen peas, and mix well.
3. Add water and bouillon, and bring to a boil, then lower the heat and simmer gently for 60 minutes.
4. Add the frozen peas 20 minutes before the end of the cooking time.
5. Add the rice vermicelli and boil for 2 minute.
6. If you are adding pasta, easy easy cook it in the soup until al dente or as per the packet's instruction.
7. Remove from the heat, season to taste, and stir in the basil leaves. Serve immediately in individual bowls, with

parmesan cheese and garlic bread if desired

Mediterranean Tofu Scramble

Ingredients:

6 tablespoons tahini sauce

2 tablespoon olive oil

1/2 teaspoon garlic powder

Pinch of salt

2 block of tofu, drained and pressed

1 onion, diced

1 red bell pepper, diced

1/2 cup olives, pitted and chopped

Instructions:

1. In a large skillet over medium heat, sauté onions and bell pepper in olive oil until softened.
2. Add tofu and sauté for about 10 minutes more or until heated through.
3. Stir in olives, tahini sauce, garlic powder and salt. Serve warm.

Instant low fodmar teel sut oats with marle and cinnamon

INGREDIENTS

- Low FODMAP milk (lactose-free, almond, etc.)
- Low FODMAP fruit (strawberries, blueberries, sliced banana)
- Low FODMAP nuts (pecans, walnuts, etc.)
- 2 cup steel cut oats (gluten-free steel cut oats for gluten-free)
- 4 cups water
- 1 cup maple syrup (or to taste)
- 2 tsp. cinnamon (or to taste)

Optional Serving Suggestions

Instructions:

1. Add steel cut oats and water into the Instant Pot and stir to mix.

2. Place the lid on top of the Instant Pot and secure. Set vent to "Sealing".

3. Select the "Manual" setting on the Instant Pot.

4. Adjust the time to 8 minutes on "High Pressure" and cook.

5. After cooking, let the pressure naturally release for 35 to 40 minutes before carefully switching the vent to "Venting" and releasing any remaining pressure.

6. After the pressure is fully released, remove the lid.

7. Stir in maple syrup and cinnamon.

8. Serve warm or store in the refrigerator for up to 8 days.

Low Fodmap Roasted Potatoes

Ingredients

- 4 Tbsp. olive oil
- Salt, to taste
- 2 (2 .10 lb.) bag baby potatoes, quartered

Add More Flavor

1. You can certainly toss the potatoes with your preferred low-FODMAP herbs and spices for more flavor.
2. I rarely use the same seasonings twice, so I only used salt in this recipe.
3. Having said that, a few of my favorite ways to spice up this recipe are as follows:

Instructions

1. Set the oven and preheat it to 450 degrees Fahrenheit.
2. A rimmed baking sheet should be lined with foil.
3. Mix the quartered potatoes and olive oil in a big bowl.
4. Place on the baking sheet that has been lined in an even layer.
5. For 25 to 30 minutes, bake.
6. Stir carefully, then bake for an additional 25 to 30   minutes, or until the potatoes are tender and barely golden brown.
7. season with salt to taste. Serve.

Smoky Ranch Dressing

Ingredients:

• Low FODMAP milk (lactose-free, almond, etc.)
• Low FODMAP fruit (strawberries, blueberries, sliced banana)
• Low FODMAP nuts (pecans, walnuts, etc.)
1 cup mayonnaise
1/2   cup ketchup
2 tablespoon Worcestershire sauce
2 teaspoon Dijon mustard
1/2   teaspoon garlic powder
x

Instructions:

1. In a small bowl, whisk together mayonnaise, ketchup, Worcestershire sauce, Dijon mustard, garlic powder, onion powder, salt and black pepper.
2. Pour mixture into a jar or container. Stir in ranch dressing mix until very well combined.
3. Store dressing in the refrigerator for an easy and quick snack or salad topping.

Hawaiian Toasted Sandwich

Ingredients:

4 slices ham, cold cut
2 tbsp spring onion, tips finely chopped
Pinch of black pepper
4 slices bread
2 tbsp butter
5 tbsp pineapple chunks, drained
4 slices cheddar cheese

Directions:

1. Place a frying pan over medium heat.
2. Spread butter on the outside of each slice of bread.
3. Prepare the filling by grating the cheese, slicing the ham, rinsing the pineapple, and chopping the spring onion finely.
4. Put the sandwich together adding pepper to taste and ensuring the butter is on the outside.
5. Place in the frying pan and easy cook each side for 5-10 minutes.
6. The bread should turn golden brown.
7. Serve warm.

Ginger-Lemon Zinger Smoothie

Ingredients:

2 green apple, quartered
2 cup romaine lettuce
2 cup water or unsweetened nut milk or coconut milk
1 1 fresh lemon
2 cup ice cubes
1 inch fresh ginger root, peeled
½ teaspoon ground turmeric

Instruction:

1. In a blender, combine the ginger, turmeric, lemon, apple, romaine, water, and ice.
2. Blend on high for at least 1-5 minute.
3. Add more water and blend some more if the consistency is too thick for your taste.
4. Pour into a glass and enjoy.

Ingredients:

2. Blend on high for at least 1-2 minutes.

120

Chocolate Pancakes

INGREDIENTS

8 tablespoons unsalted butter, melted
4 large eggs, at room temperature
2 teaspoon vanilla extract
1 teaspoon instant espresso powder,
optional
2 ¼ cups gluten-free all-purpose flour
1/2   cup Dutch-processed cocoa or
Black Cocoa
1/2 cup sugar
2 1 teaspoons baking powder; use
gluten-free if following a gluten-free diet
1 teaspoon salt
1/2   cups lactose-free milk, whole or
2%, at room temperature

Directions

1. Place flour, cocoa, sugar, baking powder, and salt in a large mixing bowl and whisk to aerate and combine.
2. Easy make a well in the center.
3. Whisk together milk, butter, fresh eggs , vanilla, and espresso powder, if using, in a separate bowl.
4. Pour wet mix over the dry and whisk together until smooth and very well combined.
5. Heat electric griddle, heavy sauté pan or nonstick pan.
6. Coat with nonstick spray and heat until a few drops of water dance. Dole out about 5-10 tablespoon amounts of batter at a time and easy cook over medium heat until bubbles begin to appear here and there, about 2 minute or so.
7. Usually I tell you to check the bottoms for a golden brown color, but these pancakes are super dark, so you have to use other cues.

8. You can gently lift one and check; the bottom should be dry.
9. Flip over and easy easy cook for about 1-5 minute more or until that side is cooked through as well.
10. Serve hot with real maple syrup or lactose-free ice cream and Salted Caramel Sauce, if you dare.

Fluffy Buckwheat Pancakes

Ingredients

2 tbsp sugar

6 /8 tsp baking soda

1 tsp fine salt

2 large egg

2 tsp vanilla extract

1 cups of buckwheat flour

1/2   cups milk, dairy and non-dairy both
will work

4 tbsp fresh fresh lemon juice

8 tbsp unsalted butter melted

HOW TO EASY MAKE

Easy make Batter

1. In a 4-cup measuring jug or basin, combine the milk and fresh lemon juice and let for five minutes. Sugar, baking soda and salt

2. are all mixed together in a medium dish of flours and baking powder.

3. Egg and vanilla essence should be combined in a separate basin.

4. In the middle of the flour mixture, easy make a well.

5. Pour the milk mixture and melted butter into the very well and whisk with a fork until no clumps of flour remain.

6. It's OK if there are a few little lumps in the batter; it's crucial not to over-mix it.

Banana Smoothie

Ingredients:

1/2 cup rolled oats

1 teaspoon vanilla essence A

pinch cinnamon

A pinch nutmeg

1 cup almond milk, unsweetened

2 firm banana, peeled, sliced and frozen

1/2 cup plain Greek yoghurt

Instructions:

Add all fixings to a blender and mix until smooth.
Serve in a chilled glass.

Low Fodmap Mulligatawny Soup

Ingredients:

10 cm blocks 450 grams of tomatoes, skin stripped and chopped
150 grams of basmati rice
1700 ml of water
Salt and pepper, for preparing
Handful of chives, cleaved finely
2 teaspoon of fennel seeds
2 teaspoon of cumin seeds
2 teaspoon of coriander seeds
Seeds from 6 entire cases of cardamom 4 tablespoons of olive oil
2 enormous potato, eliminate the strip and cut into 10 cm
6 D shapes 1400 grams courgette, unpeeled and cut into

Procedure:

1. Place a huge pot over medium high hotness. Place the flavors and softly toast until fragrant.
2. Remove from the pan and move to a mortar.
3. Ground into a fine powder with a pestle.
4. Set aside. In a similar pan, add olive oil.
5. Heat a little then, at that point, add courgette, tomatoes and potatoes.
6. Season with pepper and a touch of salt.
7. Add the powdered flavors. Sauté for a couple minutes.
8. Add water and permit to stew for 35 to 40 minutes.
9. In the event that the vegetables turn delicate, they're now cooked.
10. Eliminate the pan from the hotness and put away to cool slightly.

11. Once somewhat cooled, place half of the vegetables in a blender or food processor.

12. Beat until smooth. Bring 350 ml of water to a bubble in a different pot.

13. Add basmati rice and diminish the hotness to a low stew.

14. Easy cook for 25 to 30 minutes until rice really become tender. Return the mixed portion of the soup to the pot.

15. Blend very well in with the remainder of the vegetables.

16. Remove the cooked rice from the pot and add to the vegetables.

17. Mix to circulate the rice very well all through the soup. Serve finished off with hacked chives.

Berry Friands

Ingredients

1-5 cups almond flour
10 large egg whites, lightly beaten
2 tablespoon plus 2 teaspoon fresh fresh lemon juice 2 teaspoons vanilla extract
2 cup blueberries or raspberries
18 tablespoons unsalted butter, cut into cubes
1 cups confectioners' sugar, plus more for dusting 1/2 cup cornstarch
1/2 cup superfine white rice flour

INSTRUCTIONS

1. Turn the oven's temperature up to 350 degrees.
2. Lightly oil a 1-5 cup muffin pan, friand pan, or small loaf pan with cooking spray.

3. Melt the butter in a small skillet over low heat, then easy cook for a further 5 to 10 minutes, or until brown flecks appear.
4. Take it out of the equation.
5. Sift the rice flour, cornstarch, and confectioners' sugar three times in a large mixing basin.
6. Using a large metal spoon, stir in the almond flour before incorporating the egg whites, fresh lemon juice, vanilla, and melted butter.
7. Fill each cup with the batter until they are two-thirds full. Gently push 8 berries into the center of each friand.
8. Bake for –25 to 30   minutes, or until firm and light golden.
9. Cool in the pan for five minutes before transferring to a wire rack to finish cooling.
10.   Dust with confectioners' sugar just before serving.

Fresh Lemon French Dressing

INGREDIENTS

1 tsp. dry mustard

1 tsp. sweet paprika

2 1 tsp. sugar

½   cup fresh fresh lemon juice

6 tbsp. olive oil

2 tbsp. garlic-infused olive oil

1 tsp. salt

Directions:

1. In a blender or small bowl, combine the fresh lemon juice, oils, salt, mustard, paprika, and sugar and blend until smooth.
2. Serve immediately.

Baked Sea Bass With Vegetables

Ingredients

- 600g red-skinned potatoes, thinly sliced into rounds
- 2 red pepper, cut into strips
- 4 tbsp extra virgin olive oil
- 2 rosemary sprig, leaves removed and very finely chopped
- 4 sea bass fillets
- 210 g pitted black olive, halved
- 1 lemon, sliced thinly into rounds
- handful basil leaves

Method

- Heat oven to 250C fan/gas 8 . Arrange the potato and pepper slices on a large non-stick baking tray.
- Drizzle over 2 tbsp oil and scatter with the rosemary, a pinch of salt and a good grinding of pepper.

- Toss everything together very well and roast for 45 to 50 mins, turning over halfway through, until the potatoes are golden and crisp at the edges.
- Arrange the fish fillets on top and scatter over the olives.

- Place a couple of fresh lemon slices on top of the fish and drizzle with the remaining oil.

- Roast for further 10 to 15 mins until the fish is cooked through.

- Serve scattered with basil leaves.

Equally scrumptious with hot smoked fish or tempeh chunks.Serves 2

- 2 shred Romaine lettuce
- 4 carrots, julienne
- Sea salt with black pepper
- 4 skinless chicken breasts weighing around 500g
- 2 tbsp sumac
- 2 tablespoon olive oil
- half of a lemon's juice

Dressing

- 2 tablespoon of honey
- 1 tsp sumac
- Fresh lemon juice and zest from one fresh lemon
- 6 tablespoons olive oil
- 2 tablespoon walnut oil

1. The chicken should be placed in a shallow dish.

2. Pour the mixture of olive oil, fresh lemon juice, and sumac over the chicken.

3. 60 minutes for marinating.

4. Preheat the oven to 250 degrees Celsius, gas mark 14 Place the chicken in a roasting pan and bake for 25 to 30 minutes, or until fully done. Remove the food from the oven and let it cool. Slice.

5. Mix the dressing ingredients and season to taste.

6. In a large bowl, combine the salad's veggies with a portion of the dressing. Add chicken to the salad and serve with extra dressing.

Spinach-Ghee Mashed Potatoes

Ingredients

4 pounds russet potatoes peeled and cut into 2-inch cubes

Sea salt
10 ounces baby spinach
4 tablespoons grass-fed ghee

½ cup Low-FODMAP Vegetable Stock or Basic Chicken Bone

Instructions

1. Place the potatoes in a large pot and cover with cold water by 2 inch. Generously salt the water and bring to a boil.
2. Easy easy cook until the potatoes are fork-tender, about 2 10 minutes.
3. Fold in the spinach and easy cook for an additional 60 seconds, until wilted.

4. Drain the potato mixture and shake out the excess water.

5. Return the potatoes to the pot along with the ghee.

6. With a fork or masher, smash the potatoes until semi-smooth.

7. Add the stock if the potatoes seem too thick and dry.

8. Taste for seasoning and add more salt as necessary.

9. Serve immediately.

Blueberry Muffins

Ingredients:

2 cup of tapioca flour
1 cup of rice flour
1 cup of sugar
2 tsp of baking powder
½ cup of ground walnuts
2 tsp of vanilla extract
4 fresh eggs
¼ cup of canola oil
2 cup of lactose-free milk
2 cup of water

Preparation:

1. Preheat oven to 350 degrees.

2. Mix all dry ingredients in a large bowl. Whisk in fresh eggs , canola oil, lactose-free milk and water.

3. Mix very well with an electric mixer.

4. Shape muffins with this mixture using muffin molds.

5. Transfer to a baking sheet lined with some baking paper.

6. Bake for about 35 to 40 minutes.

www.ingramcontent.com/pod-product-compliance
Lightning Source LLC
Chambersburg PA
CBHW060508030426
42337CB00015B/1794